NATURAL REMEDIES FOR DRY EYES AND DIGITAL EYESTRAIN FOR OFFICE WORKERS AND SENIORS

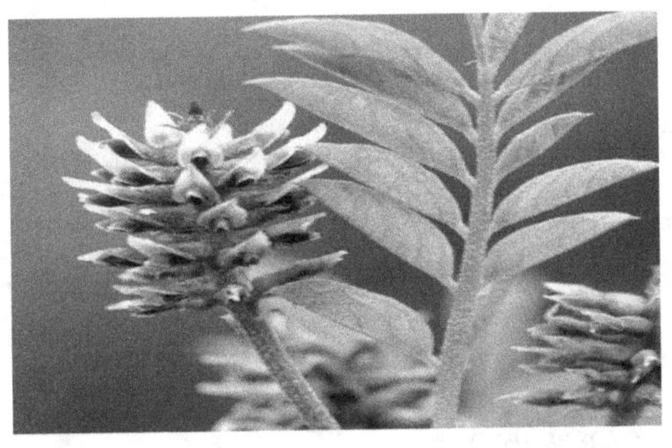

Beat Dry Eyes & Conquer Screen Strain: Proven Natural Remedies for Quick Relief for Busy Office Workers and Seniors

Dr Ikukoyi Oluwaseun Akintan

Copyright

Natural Remedies For Dry Eyes And Digital Eye Strain For Office Workers

Copyright © 2024 by Dr. Ikukoyi Oluwaseun Akintan

ISBN: 9798324590116

Dedication

This book is dedicated to the Almighty God, the giver of all good things for mankind to enjoy.

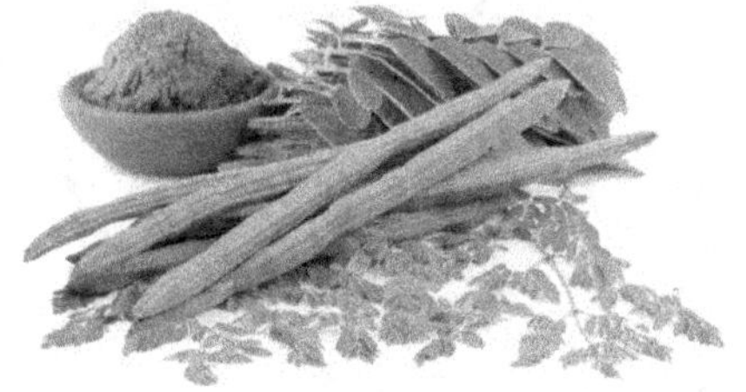

Disclaimer

This book is intended to equip you with knowledge regarding eye health. The supplied information is solely intended for educational purposes and should not be construed as medical advice. Always visit an optometrist or an ophthalmologist for diagnosis, treatment suggestions, and to address any specific eye concerns you may have.

Both the author and the publisher disclaim any liability for any accident or health issue that may arise from the utilization of the information provided.

Table of Contents

"Up to 12million Americans suffer from a disease called Dry Eye Syndrome."

-American Academy of Ophthalmology

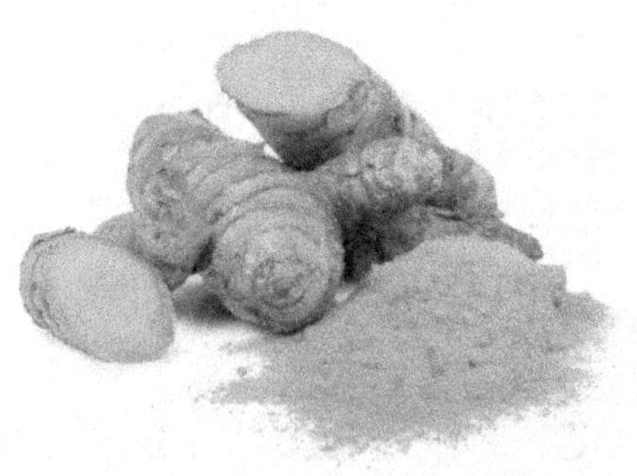

INTRODUCTION

UNDERSTANDING DRY EYES IN SENIORS: A COMMON DISCOMFORT WITH SIGNIFICANT IMPACT

Dry eyes, officially termed Dry Eye Disease (DED), are a widespread issue among seniors, affecting a considerable section of the aging population. This illness can emerge as a continuous feeling of dryness, irritation, and discomfort in the eyes, greatly reducing quality of life. Simple chores like reading, using a computer, or simply enjoying the outdoors might become a challenge.

Here, we look into the primary reasons contributing to dry eyes in seniors:

Causes of Dry Eyes in Older Adults:

Decreased Tear Production:

The lacrimal glands, positioned above the eyes, are responsible for producing tears, a crucial fluid that lubricates and protects the ocular surface. Unfortunately, tear production naturally reduces with age. Studies have demonstrated a considerable decrease in tear volume in those over 65 compared to younger adults. This drop in tear production is a crucial contributor in the development of dry eyes in elderly.

Changes in Tear Quality:

While tear volume is significant, tear quality plays an equally important impact. Tears are a complicated mixture of water, oil (lipids), and mucus. This precise formulation maintains adequate lubrication, reduces tear evaporation, and protects the eye from irritants. With aging, the content of tears might change, leading to a decrease in the oil layer. This results in tears that evaporate more quickly, failing to effectively lubricate the eye's surface and leaving it exposed to dryness.

Medical disorders:

Several age-related medical disorders are connected to an increased risk of dry eyes in seniors. These include:

Autoimmune diseases: Conditions including Sjogren's syndrome and rheumatoid arthritis can impair the lacrimal glands, resulting to decreased tear production.

Thyroid disorders: Both hyperthyroidism and hypothyroidism can lead to dry eyes.

Diabetes: Diabetic neuropathy, nerve damage induced by diabetes, can disrupt the lacrimal glands and tear production.

Drugs: Certain drugs often provided to seniors can contribute to dry eyes as a side effect. These treatments include: Antihistamines: Used for allergies, these medications can dry up the eyes as they prevent the release of histamine, a molecule that also plays a role in tear production.

Decongestants: Used for nasal congestion alleviation, these drugs can also have a drying effect on the eyes.

Diuretics: Medications used to treat high blood pressure can sometimes contribute to dry eyes by increasing urine and potentially leading to dehydration.

Blood pressure drugs: Some forms of blood pressure medications, such as beta-blockers, can also have drying effects on the eye.

Symptoms of Dry Eyes:

Seniors with dry eyes may encounter a number of symptoms, often causing discomfort and interfering with regular activities. These symptoms can include:

- A grainy or scratchy sensation in the eyes, commonly characterized as feeling like sand is present.

- Burning or stinging feeling in the eyes.

- Redness of the eye, often seeming bloodshot.

- Blurred vision, especially visible during prolonged reading or computer use.

- Sensitivity to light, causing discomfort in bright situations.

- Excessive tearing (paradoxical tearing): This may seem illogical, but the body's attempt to overcompensate for inadequate lubrication can lead to excessive tear production, which soon evaporates and fails to wet the eyes effectively.

The Importance of Eye Lubrication for Seniors:

Maintaining sufficient eye lubrication is crucial for good eye health, especially for seniors. Tears play a key function in:

Lubricating the cornea: Tears provide a smooth, moist surface for the cornea, the transparent outer layer of the eye, enabling for pleasant blinking and eye movement [10]. This lubrication enables clean vision and protects the cornea from friction.

Washing away dust, debris, and pathogens: Tears operate as a natural defensive system, washing away dust, debris, and pathogens that may enter the eye. This helps prevent infections and keeps the ocular surface healthy.

Maintaining a healthy ocular surface: Tears contribute to maintaining a healthy environment on the surface of the eye. They nourish the cornea and provide excellent eyesight.

It is important for seniors and their caretakers to understand the factors that contribute to dry eyes and how to preserve eye health.

References:

1. Ljubimov, V. I., & Mochalova, O. V. (2018). Age-related changes in tear function in healthy adults. Ophthalmic Research, 59(2), 142-147.

2. Nicholson, D. P., Murphy, P. J., Bradley, M., Lindgren, G., & Gao, J. (2017). The tear film in dry eye disease: A lipid oasis

in a tear desert. Experimental Eye Research, 159, 176-186.

3. American Academy of Ophthalmology. (2023, May 17). Dry eye.

4. National Eye Institute. (n.d.). Dry Eyes. https://www.studystack.com/flashcard-932317

"Prioritize your eye health, keep your world in proper focus, invest in your well-being, and reap the rewards of a lifetime of clear vision."

— Robert M. Kershner, MD, MS, FACS

CHAPTER ONE

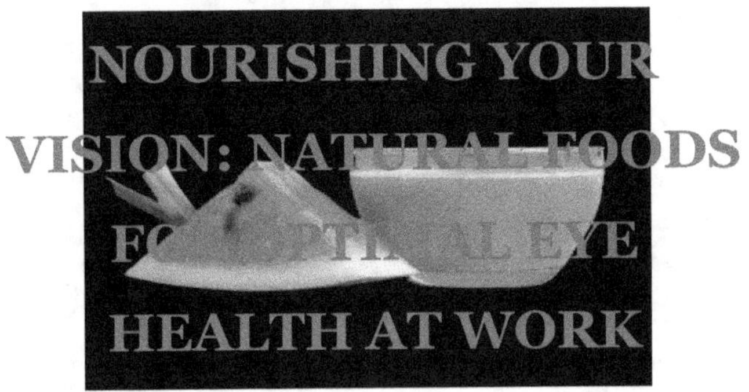

Long hours spent staring at computer screens can take a toll on your eyes. Dryness, irritability, and tension are all typical concerns among office workers. But what you put on your plate can substantially affect your eye health and visual comfort. This chapter covers the importance of a balanced diet for eye health and includes a guide on adding key nutrients into your workday meals and snacks.

The Link Between Diet and Eye Health:

The eyes rely on a range of nutrients to function correctly. A well-balanced diet rich in certain vitamins, minerals, and antioxidants can help protect your eyes from age-related macular degeneration (AMD), cataracts, and other eye problems [1].

Essential Nutrients for Eye Health:

Lutein and Zeaxanthin: These carotenoids found in leafy green foods like kale, spinach, and collard greens, accumulate in the macula, the core region of the retina responsible for clear central vision. They serve as antioxidants, protecting the eyes from light damage [1].

Vitamin A: Essential for preserving healthy vision, Vitamin A is found in orange and yellow fruits and vegetables like carrots, sweet potatoes, and melons. It also has a function in night vision [2].

Vitamin C: A potent antioxidant, Vitamin C found in citrus fruits, berries, and tomatoes helps protect eye cells from injury and may lessen the development of cataracts [3].

Vitamin E: Another vital antioxidant, Vitamin E found in nuts, peanuts, and avocados, helps prevent free radical damage in the eyes [4].

Omega-3 Fatty Acids: These healthy fats found in fatty fish like salmon, tuna, and sardines, may play a role in lowering dry eye symptoms and boosting general eye health [5].

Incorporating Eye-Healthy Foods Into Your Workday:

Start Your Day with a Colorful Plate: Include a variety of brightly colored fruits and vegetables in your breakfast for a boost of lutein, zeaxanthin, and Vitamin C.

Snack Smart: Opt for healthy snacks like nuts, seeds, or dried fruits throughout the day to keep your energy levels up and give critical nutrients for your eyes.

Pack a Nutritious Lunch: Prepare your lunch at home to ensure you have control over the food. Include a leafy green salad, lean protein source, and colorful veggies for a balanced and eye-healthy dinner.

Stay Hydrated: Drinking enough of water throughout the day helps keep your eyes lubricated and prevents dry eye symptoms.

Carry a reusable water bottle and aim to sip water regularly.

Reference

1. Khadivzadeh, S., Sun, D., Margolis, LJ., Tsao, H., & Hankinson, SE. (2016). Dietary lutein and zeaxanthin and the risk of age-related macular degeneration: A systematic review and meta-analysis. Ophthalmology, 123(3), 796-805.

https://doi.org/10.1016/j.ophtha.2015.11.023

2. National Institutes of Health. (2021, September 29). Vitamin A. https://ods.od.nih.gov/

3. Eye Diseases Prevalence Research Group. (2007). Dietary factors and the incidence of age-related maculopathy: The AREDS Report No. 3. Archives of Ophthalmology, 115(11), 1633-1643.

4. National Eye Institute. (n.d.) Facts about vitamins and eye health. https://www.nei.nih.gov/about/news-and-events/news/nih-study-provides-clarity-supplements-protection-against-blinding-eye-disease

5. Dry Eye Working Group. (2016). The role of dietary omega-3 fatty acids in dry eye disease. Ocular Surface, 14(3), 439-453.

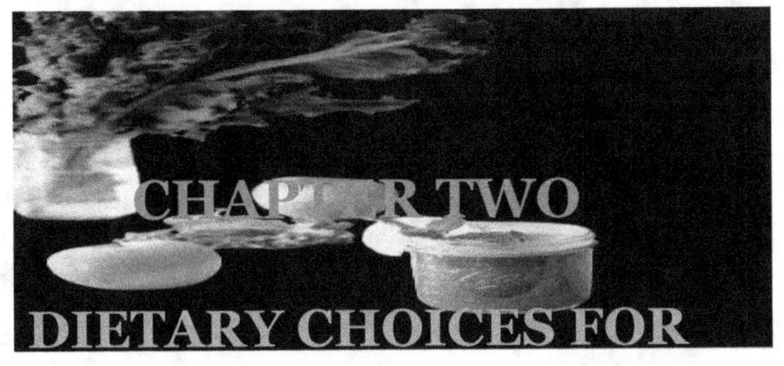

EYE HEALTH IN SENIORS

While dry eyes can be a painful effect of aging, some dietary choices might contribute to improved eye health and potentially ease some of the discomfort associated with dry eyes in seniors. Here, we study how particular nutrients can play a role in enhancing tear quality and general eye health:

Omega-3 Fatty Acids:

Importance: Omega-3 fatty acids, particularly EPA and DHA, are crucial for maintaining healthy cell membranes throughout the body, including those in the lacrimal glands [1]. Studies suggest that enough Omega-3 intake may assist enhance tear production and improve tear quality [2].

Dietary Sources: Fatty fish (salmon, tuna, mackerel) [3].

Flaxseeds with chia seeds [4].

Walnuts and hemp seeds [5].

Vitamins A & E:

Importance: Vitamins A and E are potent antioxidants that play a critical role in protecting the eye from oxidative damage caused by free radicals. This damage can contribute to dry eyes and age-related macular degeneration (AMD) [6].

Vitamin A: Essential for maintaining a healthy cornea and tear production [7].

Vitamin E: Helps prevent cell membranes from free radical damage in the eye [8].

Dietary Sources:

Vitamin A: Orange and yellow veggies (carrots, sweet potatoes), leafy green vegetables (spinach, kale), eggs [9].

Vitamin E: Nuts and seeds (almonds, sunflower seeds), vegetable oils (olive oil, avocado oil) [10].

Staying Hydrated:

Importance: Dehydration might increase dry eye symptoms. Proper hydration is critical for maintaining the water content of tears and guaranteeing their efficiency in lubricating the eye [11].

Recommendation: Aim for appropriate water consumption throughout the day. The exact amount can vary depending on individual characteristics, but a basic rule is to drink eight glasses of water every day [12].

Sample Meal Plan:

Here's a sample meal plan high in the nutrients listed above, which might be a starting point for seniors wishing to add eye-healthy choices into their diet:

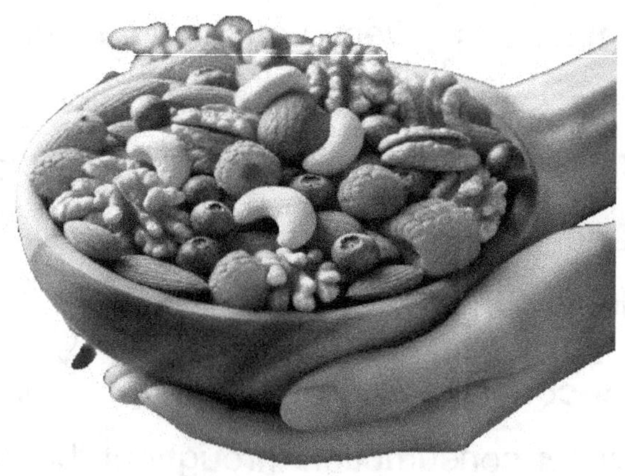

Meal Plan 1:

Breakfast: Omega-3 scrambled eggs with spinach and whole-wheat toast, alongside a glass of orange juice (great source of Vitamin A).

Lunch: Grilled salmon with a side of roasted sweet potatoes (high in Vitamin A) and steamed broccoli (excellent source of Vitamin A and C).

Snack: Handful of nuts and a cup of berries (antioxidants).

Dinner: Chicken stir-fry with colorful veggies (carrots, bell peppers) and brown rice, drizzled with olive oil (Vitamin E).

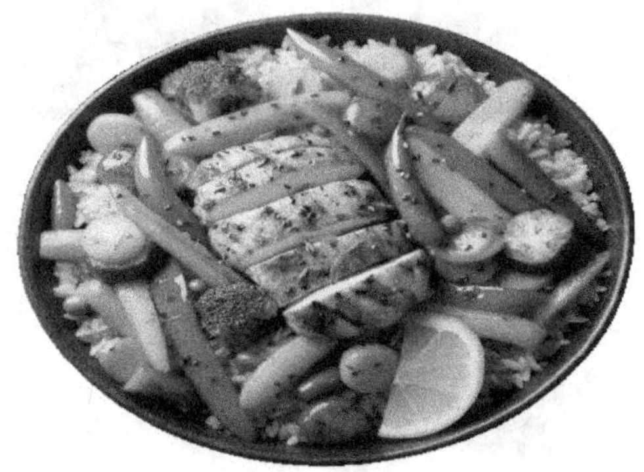

Meal Plan 2:

Breakfast: Greek yogurt with berries and a sprinkling of chopped walnuts (protein, antioxidants)

Lunch: Lentil soup with whole-grain bread and a side salad with olive oil vinaigrette (protein, fiber, omega-3s)

Snack: Cottage cheese with sliced pineapple (protein, Vitamin C)

Dinner: Baked chicken breast with roasted Brussels sprouts and quinoa (protein, Vitamin K)

Meal Plan 3:

Breakfast: Oatmeal with sliced banana and a drizzle of honey (fiber, potassium)

Lunch: Tuna salad sandwich on whole-wheat bread with a side of young carrots (protein, Vitamin A)

Snack: Handful of assorted nuts and dried cranberries (healthy fats, antioxidants)

Dinner: Salmon with roasted sweet potato segments and steamed asparagus (omega-3s, Vitamin A, Vitamin C)

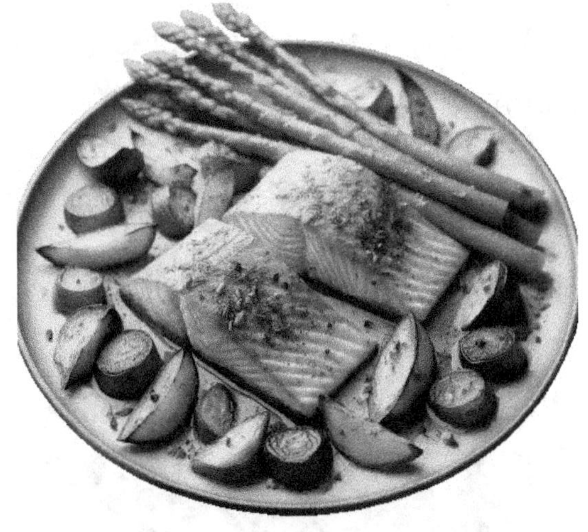

Meal Plan 4:

Breakfast: Scrambled eggs with spinach and whole-wheat crostini, alongside a glass of tomato juice (protein, Vitamin C, lycopene)

Lunch: Black bean burger on a whole-wheat bun with a side salad with avocado dressing (protein, healthful fats)

Snack: Pear with a dollop of almond butter (fiber, Vitamin C, healthful fats)

Dinner: Turkey chili with brown rice and a side of chopped fresh vegetables (protein, fiber, Vitamin C)

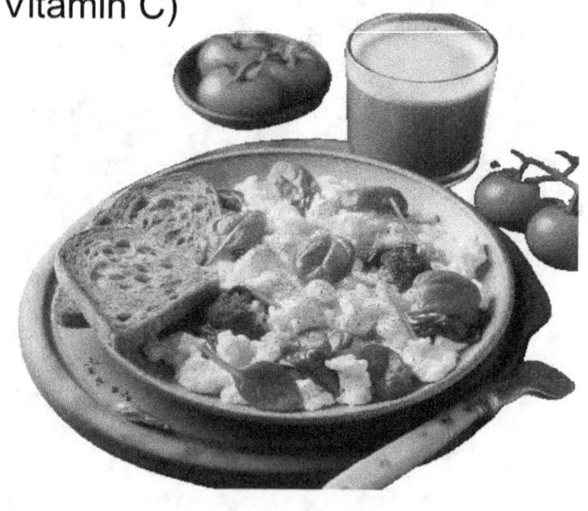

Meal Plan 5:

Breakfast: Whole-wheat crêpes with blueberries and a drizzle of maple syrup (fiber, antioxidants)

Lunch: Chicken Caesar salad with whole-wheat croutons (protein, Vitamin K)

Snack: Edamame pods (protein, Vitamin K)

Dinner: Vegetarian stir-fry with tofu, colorful vegetables (bell peppers, broccoli), and brown rice (protein, antioxidants)

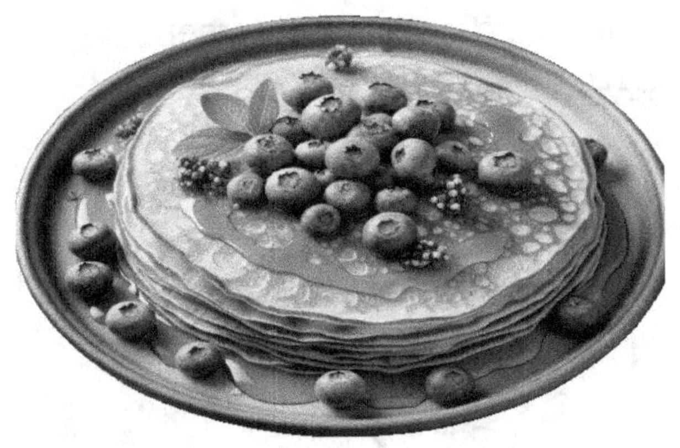

Meal Plan 6:

Breakfast: Smoothie made with Greek yogurt, spinach, banana, and a dash of orange juice (protein, Vitamin C, potassium)

Lunch: Chickpea salad sandwich on whole-wheat bread with a side of cucumber slices (protein, fiber)

Snack: Apple slices with a sprinkling of cinnamon (fiber, Vitamin C)

Dinner: Baked cod with roasted sweet potato and steamed green asparagus (protein, Vitamin A)

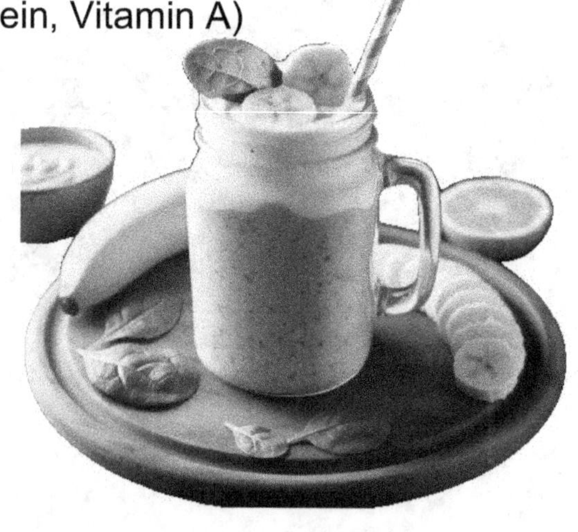

Meal Plan 7:

Breakfast: Whole-wheat waffles with scrambled eggs and a side of fruit salad (protein, fiber, vitamins)

Lunch: Lentil and vegetable soup with whole-grain crackers (protein, fiber)

Snack: Cottage cheese with diced peaches (protein, Vitamin C)

Dinner: Chicken stir-fry with broccoli, carrots, and brown rice (protein, Vitamin A)

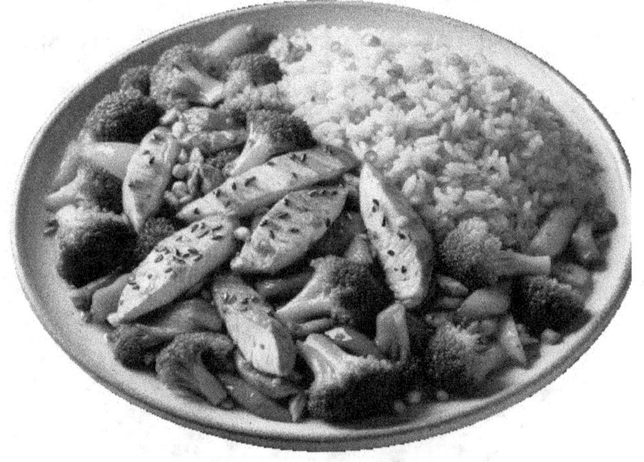

Meal Plan 8:

Breakfast: Whole-wheat toast with avocado slices and a sprinkle of everything bagel seasoning (healthy lipids, fiber)

Lunch: Chicken breast sandwich on whole-wheat bread with lettuce, tomato, and avocado (protein, healthy lipids)

Snack: Handful of dried apricots and almonds (fiber, Vitamin A, healthful fats)

Dinner: Baked salmon with roasted Brussels sprouts and quinoa (protein, omega-3s, fiber)

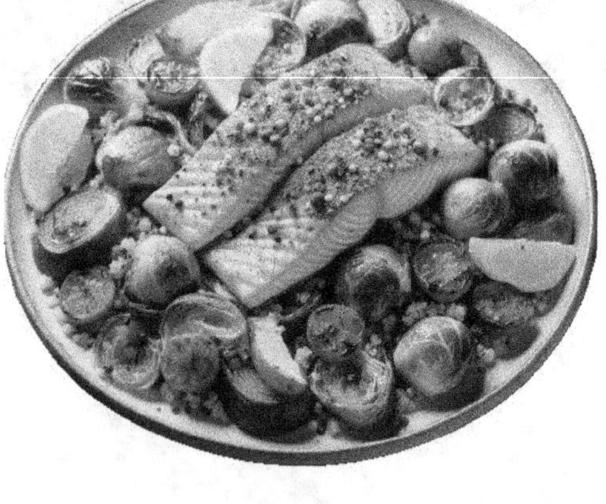

Meal Plan 9:

Breakfast: Whole-wheat English muffin with scrambling eggs and a side of sliced tomato (protein, Vitamin C)

Lunch: Tuna salad with diced vegetables (celery, onion) on a bed of romaine lettuce (protein, fiber)

Snack: Greek yogurt with a dusting of granola and berries (protein, antioxidants)

Dinner: Turkey chili with whole-wheat bread and a side salad with vinaigrette dressing (protein, fiber, Vitamin C)

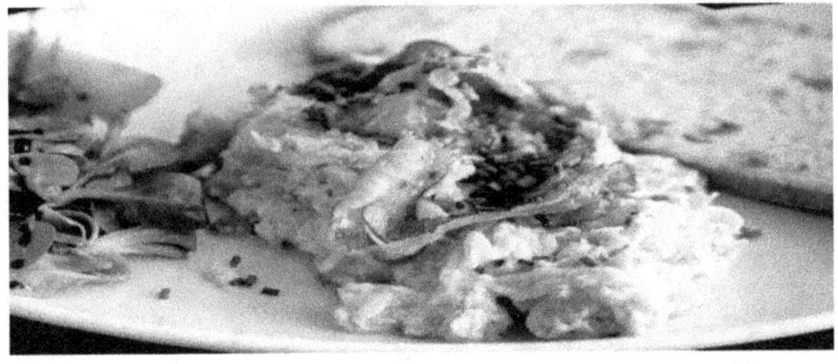

Meal Plan 10:

Breakfast: Oatmeal with chopped walnuts and a drizzle of honey (fiber, healthful fats)

Lunch: Chicken Caesar salad with whole-wheat croutons (protein, Vitamin K)

Snack: Cottage cheese with diced peaches (protein, Vitamin C)

Dinner: Shrimp stir-fry with colorful vegetables (broccoli, peppers) and brown rice (protein, antioxidants)

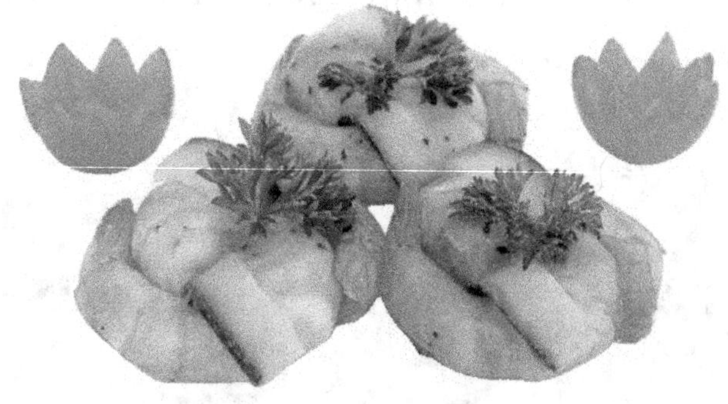

Meal Plan 11:

Breakfast: Smoothie made with Greek yogurt, spinach, banana, and a dash of orange juice (protein, Vitamin C, potassium)

Lunch: Chicken breast sandwich on whole-wheat bread with lettuce, tomato, and avocado (protein, healthful fats)

Snack: Handful of assorted nuts and dried cranberries (healthy fats, antioxidants)

Dinner: Baked cod with roasted sweet potato and steamed asparagus (protein, Vitamin A, Vitamin C)

Meal Plan 12

Breakfast: Greek yogurt with berries, granola, and a sprinkle of chopped almonds (protein, antioxidants, Vitamin E)

Lunch: Salmon with roasted Brussels sprouts and quinoa (protein, omega-3s, Vitamin K)

Snack: Handful of mixed nuts and dried cranberries (healthy fats, antioxidants)

Dinner: Chicken stir-fry with colorful vegetables (bell peppers, broccoli) and brown rice (protein, antioxidants)

Remember, these are just examples, and you can customize them based on your preferences and dietary

Additional Tips:

Limit processed meals and sugary drinks: These might contribute to inflammation in the body, perhaps increasing dry eye problems.

Consult with a healthcare professional: Discuss dietary modifications with your doctor or a certified dietitian to ensure they correspond with your overall health needs.

By following these dietary habits and keeping a healthy lifestyle, seniors might potentially enhance their eye health and experience relief from dry eye problems.

References:

1.	Graue, T., & Grünwald, J. (2017). Potential of omega-3 fatty acids in managing dry eye disease. Ophthalmologica, 238(1), 1-8. https://pubmed.ncbi.nlm.nih.gov/19227095/

2.   Liu, X. Z., & Zhu, L. (2017). The role of omega-3 polyunsaturated fatty acids in the treatment of dry eye disease. Ophthalmic Reviews, 9(2), 113-118. https://www.ncbi.nlm.nih.gov/pmc/articles/PMC9744874/

3.   National Institutes of Health. (2020, September 24). Omega-3 Fatty Acids. https://pubmed.ncbi.nlm.nih.gov/19227095/

4.   Mayo Clinic. (2020, August 21). Flaxseed: A safety consideration. https://newsnetwork.mayoclinic.org/discussion/mayo-clinic-q-and-a-flaxseed-a-nutritional-powerhouse/

5.   Cleveland Clinic. (2021, June 24). What are some good sources of omega-3 fatty acids? https://my.clevelandclinic.org/health/drugs/18818-fish-oil-omega-3-fatty-acids-capsules-otc

6.   National Eye Institute. (n.d.). Facts About Age-Related Macular Degeneration

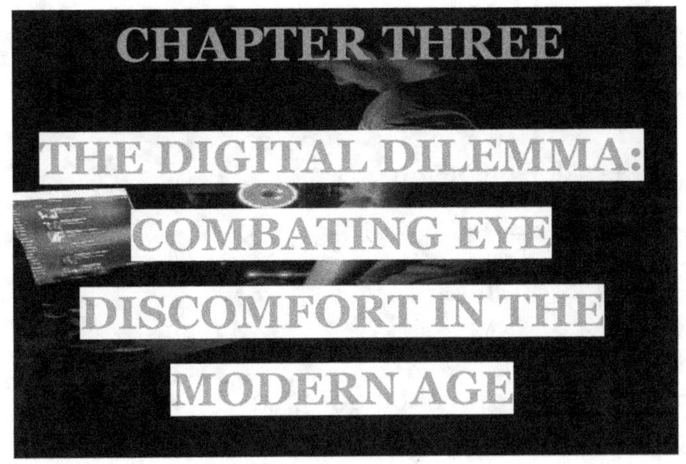

Our digital world offers unlimited options for connection, information, and enjoyment. However, prolonged screen time can come at a cost - eye strain. This chapter discusses the issues of digital eye strain and goes into practical techniques to minimize discomfort and improve healthy vision.

Understanding Digital Eye Strain:

Digital eye strain (DES), often known as computer vision syndrome, is a combination of eye and vision-related disorders reported by those who use digital devices for extended durations [1]. Common symptoms include:

- Blurred vision
- Dry eyes
- Eye fatigue
- Headaches
- Neck and shoulder pain

These symptoms result from numerous reasons related with digital gadget use:

Reduced Blinking: When interested on a screen, blinking frequency automatically decreases. Blinking is crucial for moisturizing the eyes and maintaining a healthy tear film [2].

Blue Light Exposure: Digital devices generate blue light, which can lead to eye strain and fatigue [3].

Poor Posture and Ergonomics: Improper viewing distance, screen orientation, and overall body posture while using digital devices can contribute to muscle tension and discomfort in the eyes, neck, and shoulders.

Combating the Digital Dilemma:

Fortunately, there are numerous practical measures you may apply to minimize digital eye strain and increase eye comfort:

Manage Screen Time:

Excessive screen time from computers, tablets, and smartphones can contribute to dry eyes. Here are some tips:

The 20-20-20 Rule:

Every 20 minutes, look away from the screen for 20 seconds and focus on an object 20 feet away. This helps relax the eyes and allows them to re-lubricate.

Adjust Screen Brightness and Positioning:

Reduce screen brightness to a comfortable level and adjust the screen position to minimize glare.

Practical Tips on Minimizing Glare Through Screen Positioning:

Glare on your screen can contribute considerably to dry eye problems and overall eye strain. Here are some practical advice on how to change your screen position to prevent glare:

Tilt Your Screen: The ideal screen position is slightly below eye level. This decreases the need to raise your eyelids as high, promoting improved tear evaporation and lubrication.

A monitor stand or adjustable arm allows you to alter the tilt for best viewing comfort.

Adjust Room Lighting: Minimize overhead lighting immediately reflecting on your computer. Opt for indirect lighting or task lamps that brighten your desk without causing a glare on the screen.

Consider using natural light if positioned properly to avoid direct sunlight falling on the screen.

Reduce Screen Brightness: Adjust your screen brightness to a reasonable level that enables clear visibility without appearing excessively bright. This can be done using the display settings or operating system controls.

Dimming the room lights further can assist balance the screen brightness for a more comfortable viewing experience.

Anti-Glare Screen Protectors: Consider putting an anti-glare screen protector on your device. This diffuses light reflection and decreases glare effectively.

Position Yourself Away From Windows: If possible, avoid sitting directly in front of a window. Natural light can generate significant glare on the screen, especially during specific times of the day.

Adjust Window Blinds or Curtains: If you can't avoid facing a window, adjust the blinds or curtains to block or deflect direct sunlight from striking your screen.

By applying these practical techniques and selecting the best screen position for your office, you may drastically minimize glare and create a more comfortable viewing environment, thereby relieving dry eye problems and eye strain.

Consider Blue Light Filtering Glasses: These glasses can help minimize exposure to blue light emitted from digital gadgets, which can lead to eye strain and dryness.

Warm Compresses: Applying warm compresses to closed eyes for 10-15 minutes a day will help stimulate the oil glands in the eyelids, resulting to enhanced tear quality.

Eyelid Hygiene: Regularly cleansing the eyelids with a gentle cleaner will remove dirt and prevent clogged oil glands, which can cause dry eyes.

Maintain a Healthy Sleep Routine: Adequate sleep is vital for general health, including eye health. Aim for 7-8 hours of sleep per night.

Artificial Tears: Over-the-counter artificial tears can provide brief relief from dry eye problems. Opt for preservative-free choices if you encounter irritation with conventional drops.

Importance of Regular Eye Exams: Regular eye exams are vital for seniors, not just for monitoring dry eyes but also for recognizing other age-related eye disorders including glaucoma and macular degeneration. Discuss your dry eye concerns with your ophthalmologist at your exams.

Remember: Consulting a healthcare professional is crucial for a proper diagnosis and specific treatment plan for dry eyes.

These recommendations are meant to enhance regular dry eye treatment, not replace it.

By following these techniques together with a nutritious diet and staying hydrated, seniors can manage their dry eye symptoms and experience greater eye comfort.

References:

1. American Academy of Ophthalmology. (2022, March 17). Computer vision syndrome.
2. National Eye Institute. (n.d.). Blinking. https://www.healthline.com/health/eye-health/eye-blinking
3. Mayo Clinic. (2020, August 21). Blue light and your eyes. https://newsnetwork.mayoclinic.org/discussion/mayo-clinic-q-and-a-are-blue-light-blocking-glasses-a-must-have/
4. American Optometric Association. (2020, July 21). Digital eye strain. https://www.ncbi.nlm.nih.gov/pmc/articles/PMC9434525/
5. The College of Optometrists. (2021, June 21). Computer vision syndrome.

https://www.college-
optometrists.org/professional-
development/college-
journals/optometry-in-practice/all-oip-
articles/volume-17,-issue-1/2016-02-
computervisionsyndrome_a-k-a-
digitaleyestr

6. National Institute of Environmental
    Health Sciences. (n.d.) Light and Your
    Health.
    https://www.gersteineye.com/blog/2018/
    08/how-does-bright-light-affect-your-
    vision/

7. American Academy of Ophthalmology.
    (2023, May 19). Dry eyes.
    https://www.aao.org/eye-
    health/treatments/dry-eye-treatment

8. Mayo Clinic. (2020, August 21).
    Computer eye strain.

9. Screen protectors: A comprehensive
    guide (2023, January 20). TechRadar.

10. American Academy of Ophthalmology. (2022, March 17). Computer vision syndrome.

11. National Sleep Foundation. (2023, March 16). How much sleep do we really need? https://www.sleepfoundation.org/how-sleep-works/how-much-sleep-do-we-really-need

12. American Academy of Ophthalmology. (2023, January 19). Comprehensive adult eye examinations.

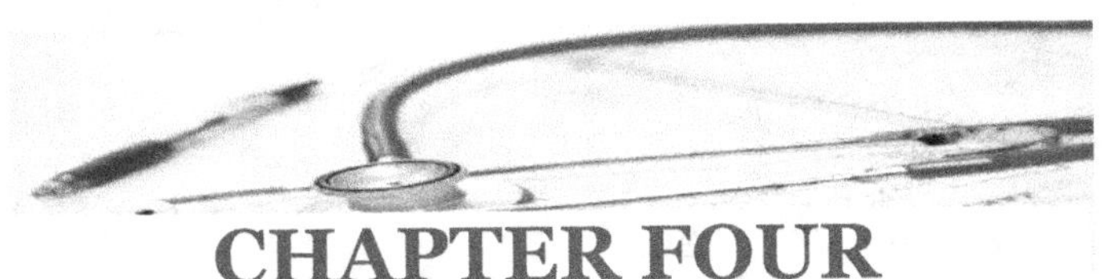

CHAPTER FOUR

WHEN TO SEEK PROFESSIONAL HELP

Your eyes are your window to the world, and preserving their health is vital for everyday living. While prioritizing a healthy diet and basic digital hygiene practices can considerably assist your vision, there are instances when obtaining professional advice from an ophthalmologist is vital. This chapter underlines the necessity of regular eye exams and examines indicators that demand prompt professional intervention.

Recognizing Persistent Dry Eyes or Worsening Vision:

Dry eye is a common ailment that can cause a range of painful symptoms, including:

- Scratchiness

- Burning feeling

- Stinging

- Redness

- Light sensitivity

- Blurred vision

While occasional dry eye symptoms are typical, especially after prolonged screen time or in dry conditions, persistent or increasing symptoms could suggest an underlying disease. If you suffer any of these symptoms for more than a few days, or if they significantly disturb your normal activities, it's crucial to contact an optometrist or ophthalmologist for a proper diagnosis and treatment plan.

Similarly, any obvious changes in your vision, such as:

- Blurred vision at any distance

- Difficulty focusing on near or far objects
- Seeing halos around lights
- Sudden flashes of light
- Loss of peripheral vision

These can be indicators of a range of eye disorders, some of which can be dangerous. Early detection and treatment are critical to prevent vision loss.

The Importance of Regular Eye Exams for Office Workers:

Even if you're not experiencing any alarming symptoms, regular eye exams are crucial for maintaining excellent eye health, especially for office workers who spend a large amount of time staring at computer screens. These exams allow your eye doctor to:

Assess your general eye health: This involves looking for early indicators of eye diseases such as glaucoma, cataracts, and macular degeneration.

Detect eyesight problems: Regular eye exams can uncover refractive defects including nearsightedness, farsightedness, or astigmatism, which can be corrected with eyeglasses or contact lenses.

Monitor eye pressure: Glaucoma, a primary cause of blindness, frequently has no early signs. Regular eye exams help your eye doctor to monitor your intraocular pressure and discover glaucoma early on when therapy is most successful.

Address any concerns: This is an ideal chance to discuss any eye-related concerns you may have, such as dry eye or digital eye strain. Your eye doctor can provide individualized advice and treatment recommendations.

The American Academy of Ophthalmology advises a full eye checkup for adults:

- At age 40, who had never had one.

- Every two to four years until age 54.

- Every one to three years for persons aged 55 to 64 years old with no serious visual issues or risk factors for eye disease.

- Every one to two years for adults aged 65 to 70 years old whether symptoms are present or not.

- Every year for adults over 70 years old [1].

Early Detection is Key:

Many eye illnesses can be adequately treated or controlled if discovered early.

Regular eye exams are a crucial preventive strategy to maintain your vision for years to come. Don't hesitate to book an appointment with your optometrist or ophthalmologist if you encounter any troubling symptoms or haven't had an eye checkup in a while.

Taking Charge of Your Eye Health: By prioritizing regular eye checkups, maintaining a healthy diet, and following excellent digital hygiene habits, you can take proactive measures towards protecting your eyesight and enjoying a lifetime of clear sight.

Reference:

American Academy of Ophthalmology. (2023, January 19). Comprehensive adult eye examinations.

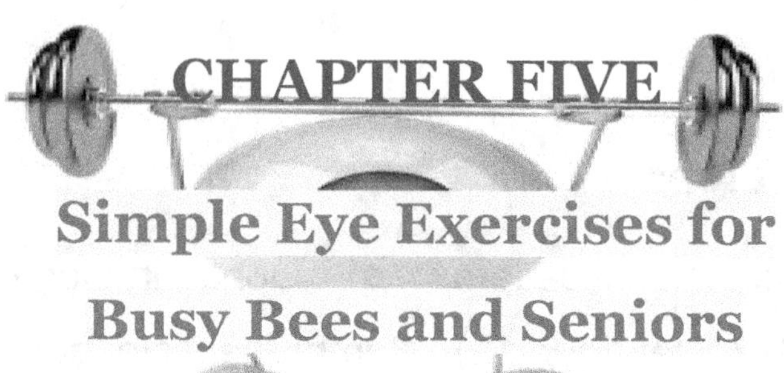

CHAPTER FIVE

Simple Eye Exercises for Busy Bees and Seniors

Beat Eye Strain During Work and Throughout the Day

Staring at digital screens for extended periods can take a toll on your eyes. Eye strain, characterized by irritation, burning, and impaired vision, is a typical complaint among office workers and anybody who spends a significant amount of time in front of computers, tablets, or smartphones. Luckily, integrating some basic eye workouts into your regular routine will considerably minimize strain and keep your eyes feeling refreshed.

The good news? These exercises are suited for both busy professionals and elderly, requiring minimal effort and time. Here are a few basic habits you may include into your workplace or throughout the day:

Simple Eye Exercises for Relaxation and Prevention of Strain

The 20-20-20 Rule:

This is a golden rule for anyone utilizing digital devices for extended periods.

- ★ Every 20 minutes, glance away from your screen for 20 seconds and gaze on an object at least 20 feet (6 meters) away.
- ★ This allows your eyes to concentrate and relax the focusing muscles.

Near-Far Focusing:

- ★ Hold your thumb at arm's length with your finger pointed upwards.
- ★ Slowly pull your thumb closer to your nose, following its movement with your eyes until it's about 3 inches away.
- ★ Then, slowly stretch your thumb back to arm's length.
- ★ Repeat this concentrating practice 10 times.

Blinking Extravaganza:

- ★ Blink rapidly for 10 seconds, squeezing your eyelids shut tightly with each blink.
- ★ Relax your eyes for 10 seconds.
- ★ Repeat this blinking sequence 3 times.

Blinking helps lubricate your eyes and spread tears evenly across the ocular surface, preventing dryness and irritation. Seniors, who may have a naturally lower blink rate, can benefit from consciously blinking more frequently throughout the day.

Eye Rolling:

- ★ Gently roll your eyes in a circular motion, 10 times in one direction,
- ★ Then, repeat 10 times in the opposite direction.

This exercise helps stretch and relax the extraocular muscles that move your eyes.

Figure of Eight

- ★ Trace an imaginary figure-eight with your eyes, horizontally.

This practice helps to control eye movement and relaxes the ocular muscles

Palming:

- ★ Rub your palms together to create warmth.
- ★ Cup your hands softly over your eyes without pressing on them.
- ★ Sit quietly for 30 seconds, allowing the warmth and darkness to ease your eyes.

Looking Up and Down:

- ★ Slowly glance up towards the ceiling,
- ★ hold for a few seconds,
- ★ then, look down to the floor.
- ★ Repeat this movement 10 times.

This exercise stretches the vertical eye muscles.

Senior-Friendly Modifications:

These exercises are generally safe for seniors, however a few tweaks can boost comfort:

Larger Print for Focusing: If focusing on a distant object (20 feet away) is problematic, utilize a larger object closer (such as a painting or clock on the wall) for the 20-20-20 rule.

Slower motions: Seniors may find slower, more controlled motions during eye rolling and looking up/down exercises more comfortable.

Seated Exercises: Most of these exercises may be done while seated, making them suitable for seniors with restricted mobility.

Remember: Consistency is crucial! Performing these exercises regularly throughout your day, even only a few minutes each, can greatly minimize eye strain and keep your vision feeling fresh.

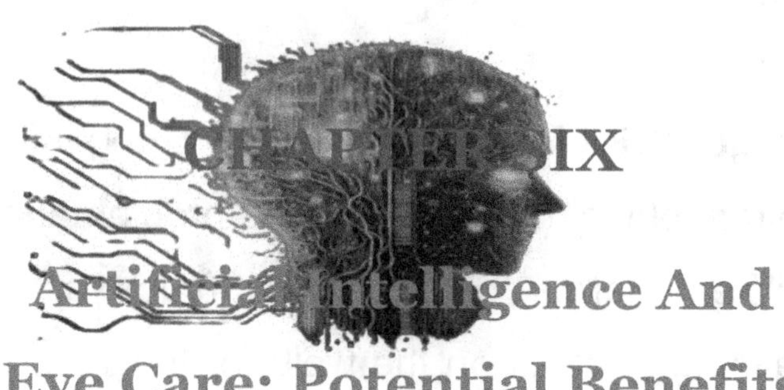

Artificial Intelligence And Eye Care: Potential Benefits And Considerations

The healthcare sector is undergoing a dramatic upheaval with the incorporation of Artificial Intelligence (AI). AI has the ability to change several parts of eye care, giving exciting opportunities for enhanced diagnosis, treatment, and overall patient experience.

Potential Applications of AI in Eye Care:

Diagnostic Assistance: AI algorithms can analyze medical images, such as retinal scans and optical coherence tomography (OCT) scans, to identify signs of eye diseases like glaucoma, diabetic retinopathy, and age-related macular degeneration (AMD) with high accuracy [1, 2]. This can assist ophthalmologists in early diagnosis and potentially lead to better treatment outcomes.

Personalized Treatment Recommendations:

AI may assess a patient's medical history, imaging data, and other criteria to produce personalized treatment suggestions. This can lead to more personalized and successful treatment options for specific needs [3].

Remote Patient Monitoring: AI-powered technology can be utilized for remote patient monitoring, allowing for early diagnosis of eye problem progression and aiding timely intervention. For instance, AI systems can analyze data from wearable devices to track intraocular pressure in glaucoma patients [4].

Development of New Ophthalmic Technologies: AI can play a major role in developing new diagnostic tools and treatment strategies for eye disorders. Advancements in AI could potentially lead to early disease identification, minimally invasive procedures, and tailored therapeutic approaches.

Considerations and Challenges of AI in Eye Care:

While AI has great promise for the future of eye care, there are critical considerations to address:

Importance of Human competence: AI should be considered as a tool to augment, not replace, the competence of ophthalmologists. The final diagnosis and treatment decisions should always lie with qualified healthcare professionals who can assess the patient's comprehensive medical history and unique circumstances.

Data Privacy and Security Concerns: The application of AI in healthcare relies significantly on patient data. Robust data security procedures are needed to preserve patient privacy and prevent any potential breaches [5].

Algorithmic Bias: AI algorithms are trained on existing datasets, and there's a risk of replicating existing biases within the data. Developers need to be cognizant of any biases in the training data to ensure AI technologies are fair and equitable for all patients [6].

The Future of AI in Eye Care

AI is still evolving in the realm of eye care. However, its potential to alter diagnostic accuracy, tailor treatment strategies, and increase patient care is evident. As AI technology continues to evolve, addressing the ethical considerations and ensuring responsible deployment will be important for reaping the full benefits of this exciting subject.

References:

1. Li, Y., Sun, L., Zheng, S., Zhao, X., Yang, G., & Cheng, J. (2020). Artificial intelligence in eye disease diagnosis. Engineering, 6(10), 1322-1331. https://doi.org/10.1016/j.eng.2020.08.013

2. Liu, X., Finn, R., Tufail, A., Aung, T., Keane, PA., & Wong, TY. (2017). Deep learning in retinal image analysis. Ophthalmology, 124(11), 1535-1544.

3. Boureau, Y., Comar, C., Villoutreix, T., Maia, BM., Haddad, N., & Palanca, A. (2017). Deep learning for retinal image segmentation. IEEE Transactions on Medical Imaging, 36(11), 2612-2624.

4. American Academy of Ophthalmology. (2023, May 19). Artificial intelligence in ophthalmology.

CHAPTER SEVEN

FINAL THOUGHTS:

Taking Charge Of Your Eye Health Naturally

Our eyes are sophisticated organs that play a significant part in how we experience the world. Protecting them and ensuring adequate vision is vital for maintaining a great quality of life. This book has studied different natural techniques you might adopt into your regular practice to maintain your eye health.

Prioritizing a Healthy Diet: As described in Chapter 1, fueling your body with vital vitamins, minerals, and antioxidants found in fruits, vegetables, and healthy fats plays a significant part in improving eye health. By including these nutrients in your diet, you can help protect your eyes from age-related macular degeneration, cataracts, and other eye disorders.

Practicing Good Digital Hygiene: Chapter 3 went into the issues of digital eye strain and presented practical solutions to combat it. Implementing the 20-20-20 rule, changing screen brightness and positioning, maintaining proper posture, and avoiding screen usage in low-light conditions can dramatically reduce eye discomfort and strain.

Regular Eye Exams: The preceding Chapter 4 underlined the significance of scheduling regular eye exams with your optometrist or ophthalmologist. These tests enable for early detection of eye disorders, identification of vision impairments, and monitoring of eye pressure. Early intervention is critical for optimizing treatment success and preventing eyesight loss.

Getting Enough Sleep: As earlier discussed in chapter 3 and elsewhere in this book, prioritizing excellent sleep is vital for general health, including eye health. When you sleep, your eyes have an opportunity to relax and restore themselves. Chronic sleep deprivation can contribute to dry eyes, impaired vision, and other eye disorders [1].

Regular Exercise: Maintaining an active lifestyle and engaging in regular physical activity can enhance your eye health in various ways. Exercise helps increase blood circulation, which is vital for delivering oxygen and nutrients to the eyes [2]. It can also help manage weight, which can be a risk factor for certain eye illnesses like diabetic retinopathy.

Managing Stress: Chronic stress can significantly affect your whole health, especially your eyes. Stress hormones can lead to dry eye symptoms and exacerbate existing eye problems. Techniques like meditation, yoga, or deep breathing techniques might help manage stress and potentially enhance eye health [3].

Taking a Holistic Approach: By embracing these natural ways, you can take ownership of your eye health and set a foundation for a lifetime of clear vision. Remember, these measures are most effective when done consistently and accompanied by regular eye exams from a trained optometrist or ophthalmologist.

Living a healthy lifestyle that prioritizes proper nutrition, digital hygiene, adequate sleep, exercise, and stress management is an investment in your long-term eye health and overall well-being.

References:

1. National Sleep Foundation. (2023, March 28). How sleep impacts your eyes and vision.

2. American Academy of Ophthalmology. (2023, January 6). Exercise and eye health.

3. National Eye Institute. (n.d.) Stress and eye health.

About the Author

Dr. Ikukoyi Oluwaseun Akintan is a seasoned optometrist with over 8 years of clinical experience. Dedicated to promoting eye health and vision wellness, Dr. Akintan combines his extensive clinical expertise with a passion for patient education and empowerment.

Through his practice, Dr. Akintan has provided comprehensive eye care to a diverse range of patients, addressing a variety of eye conditions and vision needs. His commitment to patient-centered care ensures each individual receives a thorough examination, clear explanations, and personalized treatment plans.

Dr. Akintan is a strong advocate for preventive eye care and believes in the importance of educating patients about how to maintain optimal eye health throughout their lives. This book, **"Natural Remedies for Dry Eyes and**

Digital Eyestrain for Office Workers and Seniors," is a testament to his dedication to empowering individuals to take a proactive approach to their vision.

Dr. Akintan is passionate about making a difference in the field of eye care and empowering individuals to safeguard their precious gift of sight.

www.ingramcontent.com/pod-product-compliance
Lightning Source LLC
Chambersburg PA
CBHW051910250726
48659CB00002B/583